NOURISH FOR LIFE:

"A Blueprint to living longer

Through

Smart Eating"

By

Richard A. Regan

Table of Contents

INTRODUCTION

In the quest for a long, vibrant, and fulfilling life, the significance of our daily food choices cannot be overstated. The concept of "Nourish for Life" goes far beyond the confines of mere sustenance; it embodies the profound impact that our dietary habits have on our overall well-being, health, and even our longevity. As we embark on a journey to explore the intricate relationship between nutrition and a fulfilling life, this guide will unravel the secrets, principles, and practices that can help us not only live longer but also thrive as we do so. Whether you are intrigued by the wisdom of centenarian cultures or are curious about the latest scientific findings in nutrition, "Nourish for Life" will be your compass, offering insights, guidance, and practical strategies to nourish your body, mind, and soul for the journey of a lifetime.

"Nourish for Life" is a exploration of the profound interplay between the foods we choose to eat and the quality of life we enjoy. It delves into the wisdom of cultures renowned for their exceptional longevity, revealing how their dietary patterns and lifestyle choices have unlocked the secrets to lasting health. From the Okinawans of Japan, who cherish a plant-based diet rich in vegetables and legumes, to the Mediterranean communities, Here olive oil, colorful produce, and a convivial approach to meal reign supreme, these extraordinary cultures offer profound insights into the art of nourishment.

This guide also dives into the latest scientific research on nutrition and its impact on aging. It brings together cutting-edge knowledge about the benefits of antioxidants, the role of healthy fats, and the power of mindful eating, showing us how these factors can promote wellness and vitality well into our golden years.

Additionally, "Nourish for Life" explores the significance of hydration, the importance of balance, and the potential advantages of practices like intermittent fasting, which have gained attention in the pursuit of longevity.

Whether you are seeking to enhance your dietary habits, adopt an healthier lifestyle, or simply gain a deeper understanding of the choices you make at the dinner table, this guide aims to provide a comprehensive roadmap for nourishing your way to health and longevity. So, embark on this journey with an open mind and an open palate, for "Nourish for Life" promises to reveals the extraordinary potential of food as not just sustenance but as a cornerstone of a fulfilling, vibrant, and enduring life.

CHAPTER ONE

LONGEVITY AND NUTRITION

Research has shown that diets low in energy however wealthy in vitamins, with an extra share of carbohydrates from plant resources, and limited consumption of dairy, fish, meat, and subtle ingredients may additionally enhance longevity.

Genetic, environmental, and life-style factors on the whole decide the lifespan of human beings. From these, vitamins are a key thing affecting our health, and several studies on various organisms and rodents have proven that nutrition has additionally the capability to increase lifespan.

How does nutrition affect longevity?

The extra nutritious ingredients humans ate, and the less junk ingredients they consumed, the higher their food diet scores. Researchers discovered that people who had continuously high weight-reduction nutrients have been up to 14% much less possibly to die compared to people who had always terrible diets.

What kind food promotes longevity?

One of the best diets for staying healthy and longer is still a Mediterranean diet. A high consumption of fruits, vegetables, whole grains, pulses, healthy fats from nuts, avocado, and olive oil, as well as herbs and spices, are characteristics of this diet. A couple times a week, seafood is included in it.

Why does nutrition affect a person's lifespan?

Early nutrition contributes to the development of reserves for both physical and mental function. Age-related decline is expected in later adulthood; nevertheless, those who grow healthy at birth develop biological reserves that help prevent or postpone age-related problems.

Does fasting enhance longevity?

It has been demonstrated that calorie restriction and intermittent fasting increase autophagy, promote DNA repair, guard against oxidative stress, reduce chronic inflammation, and ultimately

Secrets to longevity

Maintaining a healthy diet and regular exercise will help lengthen your life expectancy. Other factors, such as overindulging in food and excessive alcohol consumption, may also shorten your lifespan by placing you at a high risk of developing specific diseases.

Consider these keys to longevity

1. Consume healthy diets

2. Engage in regular exercise

3. Get sufficient sleep

4. Keep away from tobacco

5. Find a to manage your stress

6. Stimulate your brain

7. Be involve with social engagements

8. Pay attention to your weight

9. Regular medical check-ups

Which meals should one avoid in order to live a long life?

Our health is negatively impacted by consuming large quantities of foods high in delivered sugars and subtle carbohydrates combined with white flour, meals high in saturated or Tran's fat, and frequent consumption of processed and purple meats. The consumption of these foods should be control

CHAPTER TWO

The Longevity Blueprints

Exploring the food habits of people who live to 100 years

We can learn a lot by studying what centenarians eat. There isn't a one-size-fits-all meal plan for them. But, there are common eating patterns among them that might help the rest of us. Remember, genes, and lifestyle count too. Here's a look at what many centenarians often eat.

Eating Like the Centenarians:
Most folks living to 100 or more often stick with foods rooted in the earth. They munch on a colorful selection of fruits, vegetables, and grains. They favour beans and nuts too. These treasures from the earth are crammed full of goodies like vitamins, minerals, fiber,

and antioxidants. All of these help keep the body running smoothly.

Choosing Fresh food over Processed:
These wise individuals rarely touch run-of-the-mill, quick-fix foods like sugary treats, takeaway meals, or ready-to-eat dishes from a packet. These are usually packed with too much sugar, unhealthy fats, and unnatural additives. Such foods can leave the door open for various health problems.

Quality Protein Picks:
Meat doesn't completely disappear from the plates of the centenarians, but it's chosen wisely. Their protein pickings often include lower-fat options like fish, chicken, and occasionally a lean steak. The emphasis is often on fish, thanks to its heart and brain-boosting omega-3 fatty acids.

Drinking Alcohol Sparingly:
A good number of centenarians sip on alcohol with restraint. Red wine is a

favorite. But, too much alcohol harms your health. So, it's vital to drink reasonably.

Eating Together:

Centenarians love to have meals together. Eating with loved ones encourages good conversation and balanced meals. Smaller portions are then the natural result.

Limited Calorie Intake:

Rarely do centenarians overeat. They are careful about their meal portions. This could support a healthy weight and ward off diseases related to being overweight.

Drinking Enough Water:

Hydration is very important to overall health. This is well understood by centenarians, who drink plenty of water. They might also sip herbal teas or other beneficial drinks.

The Mediterranean Diet Influence:

In examining the diets of centenarians, we find that many of them follow dietary patterns reminiscent of the Mediterranean diet, which emphasizes the goodness of olive oil, fish, whole grains, and an abundance of fruits and vegetables. Beyond the delectable taste, this particular diet is associated with a plethora of health benefits, including a reduced risk of chronic diseases.

The Significance of Adaptation to Local Cuisine:

One noticeable trend among centenarians is their inclination toward foods that are locally sourced and deeply rooted in their region's traditions. These culinary delights often comprise a delightful medley of seasonal and fresh ingredients, each brimming with an abundance of nutrients and phytochemicals that nourish the body and invigorate the senses.

Fasting and Caloric Restriction: A Balanced Approach:

Some centenarians choose to incorporate intermittent fasting or caloric restriction into their lifestyles, having recognized the potential longevity benefits associated with these practices. However, it is crucial to approach such endeavors with caution and under the guidance of a healthcare professional. Responsible implementation of these techniques is key to optimizing the benefits they can provide.

Diet: Just One Piece of the Puzzle:

While diet undoubtedly plays a vital role in nurturing a long and healthy life, it is crucial to consider the broader spectrum of factors that contribute to overall well-being. Genetics, physical activity, mental well-being, and other lifestyle factors all intertwine to create the tapestry of longevity. Therefore, if one seeks to embrace the wisdom of the centenarian-inspired diet, consulting with a healthcare professional or registered dietitian to create a personalized plan tailored to individual needs and goals is highly recommended.

Exploring Extraordinary Cultures and their Dietary Habits:

The exploration of cultures boasting exceptional longevity offers invaluable insights into the intricate relationship between dietary patterns and a prolonged, vibrant existence. Various regions worldwide are renowned for their high concentration of centenarians, and it is fascinating to observe the shared dietary and lifestyle habits among these remarkable individuals.

Let us delve into some of these extraordinary cultures and their dietary patterns:

Okinawa, Japan: The Nourishment of Longevity:

The Okinawan diet has captivated the attention of many due to the region's impressive number of centenarians. Rich in plant-based delights, the traditional Okinawan diet prominently features a diverse array of vegetables, sweet potatoes, tofu, and seaweed. Fish and meat, while not neglected altogether, occupy a lesser space on the plate. Okinawans diligently practice portion control, seeking moderation in caloric intake. Furthermore, they place great importance on social connections and mindful eating, promoting a holistic approach to well-being.

The Mediterranean Region: A Bountiful Life Enriched by Food:

In countries like Greece, Italy, and Spain, the Mediterranean diet reigns supreme, heralded for its association with exceptional longevity. Filled to the brim with the vibrancy of fruits, vegetables, whole grains, olive oil, and moderate portions of fish, poultry, and red wine, this diet gifts its adherents with a wealth of heart-healthy fats, antioxidants, and fiber.

Sardinia, Italy: The Essence of the "Blue Zone":

The island of Sardinia, nestled within the realm of the "Blue Zones," where centenarians thrive, has its unique dietary customs. The Sardinian diet revolves around the harmonious unity of whole-grain bread, beans, lean meats, and an abundance of locally grown vegetables. A symphony of herbs graces their dishes, infusing them with delightful flavors, while red wine makes its appearance in moderation, truly capturing the essence of life's pleasures.

Ikaria, Greece: Nourishing the Body and Spirit:

Another captivating "Blue Zone," the island of Ikaria, bestows its inhabitants with remarkable longevity. Centered on whole grains, legumes, wild greens, herbs, and the nourishing embrace of olive oil, this diet provides a haven for the consumption of fish and goat dairy products in moderation. The preservation of ancient culinary wisdom is a testament to the island's dedication to nurturing both the body and spirit.

Nicoya Peninsula, Costa Rica: The Bounty of Nature's Gifts:

On the sun-drenched shores of the Nicoya Peninsula, the centenarian diet thrives on a plentiful array of vegetables, legumes, corn, and a delightful assortment of fruits such as papaya and mango. Fish and lean meats play a supporting role, while the diet's fiber-rich and antioxidant-packed profile ensures a blissful journey toward vibrant health.

Seventh-day Adventists: A Celebration of Life and Health:

The community of Seventh-day Adventists graces Loma Linda, California, and stands as a powerful symbol of longevity. Their nourishment stems from a largely plant-based diet that reveres the magnificence of fruits, vegetables, whole grains, nuts, and legumes. Often embracing vegetarian or vegan lifestyles, these individuals prioritize the adoption of healthy lifestyle choices, including regular exercise, further fortifying their path to a prolonged existence.

Hunza Valley, Pakistan: The Fountain of Health and Vitality:

Deep within the enchanting Hunza Valley resides a people renowned for their extraordinary longevity. Their diet encompasses the wonders of whole grains, fruits, vegetables, dairy products, and the occasional indulgence in small portions of meat. Moreover, the Hunza people are blessed with access to fresh, glacier-fed water, a gift that nourishes their bodies and enriches their lives.

Shared Wisdom: Building Blocks of a Long and Healthy Life:

These cultures, each with their unique dietary tapestry, converge on several significant aspects that contribute to their remarkable longevity. An unwavering focus on plant-based foods, whole grains, and the incorporation of healthy fats takes center stage. Simultaneously, cautious consumption of processed and sugary foods finds its rightful place on the sidelines. Portion control and moderate alcohol intake often punctuate their culinary practices, fostering a balanced approach to nutrition. Social connections and a love for physical activity also weave harmoniously into the fabric of their overall well-being.

It is essential to acknowledge that while diet plays an undeniable role in the longevity of these cultures, genetics, lifestyle choices, and environmental elements influence the intricate tapestry of life. Furthermore, it is important to note that the specific dietary patterns within these regions can vary, and not every individual within these populations adheres strictly to traditional diets. Nevertheless, these cultures offer us an invaluable treasure trove of lessons, urging us to embrace the benefits of a balanced, plant-centric diet, ultimately enriching our lives and illuminating the path to a long and flourishing existence.

CHAPTER THREE

The Science of Aging and Nutrition

Understanding how diet affects the aging process.

Diet plays a crucial role in the aging process, influencing various aspects of health and contributing to how our bodies age.

Lets look at some key ways in which diet affects the aging process:

Inflammation: Chronic inflammation is associated with aging and age-related diseases. Certain foods, such as those high in saturated fats, refined sugars, and processed foods, can promote inflammation. On the other hand, an anti-inflammatory diet rich in fruits, vegetables, whole grains, and omega-3 fatty acids may help reduce inflammation and support healthy aging.

Oxidative Stress: Free radicals, produced during normal cellular processes and in response to environmental factors, can cause oxidative stress, damaging cells and contributing to aging. Antioxidants found in colorful fruits and vegetables, as well as in foods like nuts and seeds, help neutralize free radicals and reduce oxidative stress.

Nutrient Intake: Adequate nutrient intake is essential for overall health and well-being. As people age, they may have changing nutritional needs and may be at risk for deficiencies in certain vitamins and minerals. A balanced and varied diet that meets these changing requirements can support healthy aging.

Bone Health: Calcium and vitamin D are crucial for maintaining bone health, and deficiencies can contribute to conditions like osteoporosis. Including dairy products, leafy greens, and fortified foods in the diet can help support bone density and reduce the risk of fractures.

Muscle Mass: Loss of muscle mass, known as sarcopenia, is common with aging. Consuming an adequate amount of protein, along with regular resistance exercises, is important for preserving muscle mass and strength.

Gut Health: The gut microbiome plays a role in various aspects of health, including digestion, immune function, and inflammation. A diet rich in fiber from fruits, vegetables, and whole grains promotes an healthy gut microbiome, which is associated with better overall health.

Weight Management: Maintaining an healthy weight is important for aging well. Obesity is associated with an increased risk of chronic diseases; while being underweight may lead to nutrient deficiencies and frailty. A balanced diet, combined with regular physical activity, contributes to weight management.

Brain Health: Certain nutrients, such as omega-3 fatty acids, antioxidants, and vitamins, are associated with brain health and cognitive function. A diet rich in these nutrients, found in fatty fish, nuts, seeds, and colorful fruits and vegetables, may help support cognitive function as people age.

Heart Health: Cardiovascular health is a key factor in aging. Diets that are high in saturated fats, sodium, and processed foods can contribute to hart diseases. On the other hand, a diet rich in fruits, vegetables, whole grains, and lean proteins can support hart health.

Hydration: Adequate hydration is important for overall health and becomes even more crucial with age. Dehydration cans lead to a range of health issues, including fatigue and impaired cognitive function. Drinking water and consuming hydrating foods, such as fruits and vegetables, supports hydration.

In summary, a well-balanced and nutrient-dense diet, along with other healthy lifestyle factors such as regular exercises and adequate sleep, can positively influence the aging process by supporting various aspects of health and reducing the risk of age-related diseases. Individual nutritional needs may vary, and it's advisable to consult with an healthcare professionals or registered dietitian for personalized advice based on specific health conditions and goals.

Understanding the role of antioxidants, inflammation, and epigenetics provides insights into the complex processes underlying longevity and aging.

Antioxidants:

Antioxidants are molecules that neutralize free radicals in the body. Free radicals are highly reactive molecules that can damage cells and contribute to aging and age-related diseases. Antioxidants are found in various foods, particularly fruits and vegetables. Examples include vitamins C and E, beta-carotene, and selenium.

A diet rich in antioxidants may help reduce oxidative stress, which is linked to aging. Some studies suggest that antioxidants may contribute to longevity by protecting cells from damage and supporting overall health.

Inflammation:

Inflammation is a natural immune response to injury or infection. However, chronic inflammation can contribute to various age-related diseases, including cardiovascular diseases, neurodegenerative disorders, and certain cancers.

Diet and lifestyle factors can influence inflammation. Foods high in refined sugars, saturated fats, and processed foods can promote inflammation, while an anti-inflammatory diet rich in fruits, vegetables, and omega-3 fatty acids can help mitigate it. Chronic inflammation is considered a hallmark of aging. Managing inflammation through a healthy lifestyle, including diet, may contribute to a longer and healthier life.

Epigenetics:

Epigenetics refers to changes in gene activity that do not involve alterations to the underlying DNA sequence. Epigenetic modifications can be influenced by environmental factors, lifestyle, and diet. Diet plays a role in epigenetic regulation. Certain nutrients, such as folate, B vitamins, and polyphenols, can influence gene expression and may impact the aging process.

Epigenetic changes can affect the expression of genes associated with aging and age-related diseases. Understanding and influencing these modifications may have implications for extending lifespan and promoting healthy aging.

Antioxidants can help counteract oxidative stress, which is often associated with inflammation. By neutralizing free radicals, antioxidants may contribute to reducing inflammation and its detrimental effects on the body.

Epigenetics and Lifestyle: Lifestyle factors, including diet, can influence epigenetic modifications. Certain dietary components, such as those with anti-inflammatory and antioxidant properties, may contribute to positive epigenetic changes associated with longevity.

Tips for Promoting Longevity:

1. Adopt an anti-inflammatory diet rich in fruits, vegetables, whole grains, and omega-3 fatty acids.

2. Consume foods high in antioxidants, including colorful fruits and vegetables, nuts, and seeds.

3. Maintain a healthy lifestyle with regular physical activity, sufficient sleep, and stress management.

4. Consider individualized approaches based on genetic factors and personalized health assessments.

While these factors play roles in longevity, it's important to recognize that aging is a complex and multifaceted process influenced by a combination of genetic, environmental, and lifestyle factors. Research in this field continues to evolve, and individual responses to interventions may vary. Consultation with healthcare professionals and registered dietitians can provide personalized guidance based on individual health needs and goals.

Nutrient-dense eating

Nutrient-dense eating involves choosing foods that provide a high concentration of essential nutrients relative to their calorie content. Prioritizing nutrient-dense foods is a key component of a healthy and balanced diet. Here are some guidelines and tips for nutrient-dense eating:

Focus on Whole Foods:

Choose whole, minimally processed foods. Whole grains, fruits, vegetables, lean proteins, and healthy fats are nutrient-dense options.

Colorful Variety:

Include a variety of colorful fruits and vegetables in your diet. Different colors often indicate the presence of various vitamins, minerals, and antioxidants.

Lean Proteins:

Opt for lean protein sources such as poultry, fish, tofu, legumes, and low-fat dairy. Protein is essential for muscle repair, immune function, and overall health.

Whole Grains:

Choose whole grains over refined grains. Examples include brown rice, quinoa, whole wheat, oats, and barley. Whole grains provide fiber, vitamins, and minerals.

Healthy Fats:

Include sources of healthy fats, such as avocados, nuts, seeds, and olive oil. These fats are important for hart health and the absorption of fat-soluble vitamins.

Limit Added Sugars:

Minimize the consumption of foods and beverages high in added sugars. Instead, satisfy sweet cravings with whole fruits.

Portion Control:

Be mindful of portion sizes to avoid overeating. Eating in moderation helps ensure a balance of nutrients without excessive calorie intake.

Hydration:

Stay hydrated with water as your primary beverages. Limit the intake of sugary drinks and excessive caffeine.

Nutrient-Rich Snacking:

Choose nutrient-dense snacks, such as fresh fruits, vegetables with hummus, Free yogurt, or a handful of nuts.

Red Food Labels:

Check food labels to understand the nutritional content of packaged foods. Look for products with fewer additives and ingredients you recognize.

Meal Planning:

Plan your meal in advance to ensure a variety of nutrient-dense foods throughout the day. This can also help you make healthier choices and avoid relying on convenience foods.

Consider Individual Needs:

Take into account your individual nutritional needs, which may vary based on factors such as age, gender, activity level, and health conditions.

Limit Processed Foods:

Processed foods often contain added sugars, unhealthy fats, and excess sodium. Choose whole, fresh foods whenever possible.

Include Dairy or Dairy Alternatives:

Incorporate sources of calcium and vitamin D, such as dairy or fortified plant-based alternatives, for bone health.

Consult with a Professional:

If you have specific dietary concerns or health conditions, consider consulting with a registered dietitian or healthcare professionals for personalized advice.

By focusing on nutrient-dense eating, you provide your body with the essential vitamins, minerals, and other compounds it needs for optimal functioning. This approach supports overall health, energy levels, and may contribute to long-term well-being.

CHAPTER FOUR

Eating for brain health

The foods we eat play a critical role in regulating everything in our bodies. From our mood to physical functioning, we know that a healthier diet can protect cognitive function while also improving other aspects of health. What we eat have positive and negative impacts on our brain.

Eating of foods that benefit the whole body is necessary, as the brain is affect by multiple bodily systems including the cardiovascular, immune, endocrine, and digestive systems. Risk factors for stroke and hart diseases are strongly connected to risk factors for dementia because the brain utilizes the energy supplied by the vasculature to function. Therefore, the types of diets that promote brain health are the some diets that are also good for better functioning of hart.

Eating for brain health involves adopting a diet that supports cognitive function, memory, and overall mental well-being. The brain, like any other organ, requires specific nutrients to function optimally.

Here are some dietary principles and tips for promoting brain health:

Omega-3 Fatty Acids:

Sources: Fatty fish (such as salmon, mackerel, and trout), flaxseeds, china seeds, walnuts, and alga-based supplements. Omega-3 fatty acids, especially DHA (docosahexaenoic acid), are crucial for brain structure and function. They support cognitive function and may have protective effects against neurodegenerative diseases.

Antioxidant-Rich Foods:

Sources: Berries (blueberries, strawberries, dark chocolate, spinach, kale, broccoli, and green tea. Antioxidants help protect the brain from oxidative stress and inflammation, which are implicated in age-related cognitive decline.

Leafy Greens and Vegetables:

Sources: Spinach, kale, broccoli, Brussels sprouts, and other colorful vegetables.

Rich in vitamins, minerals, and antioxidants, leafy greens and vegetables contribute to overall brain health by providing essential nutrients.

Whole Grains:

Sources: Quinoa, brown rice, oats, and whole what. Whole grains provide a steady supply of energy to the brain. They contain complex carbohydrates, fiber, and various nutrients that support cognitive function.

Berries:

Sources: Blueberries, strawberries, raspberries, and blackberries. Berries are rich in antioxidants and flavonoids that have been linked to improved cognitive function and may help protect the brain from age-related decline.

Nuts and Seeds:

Sources: Almonds, walnuts, flaxseeds, china seeds, and sunflower seeds. Nuts and seeds provide essential nutrients such as omega-3 fatty acids, antioxidants, and vitamin E, which support brain health.

Lean Proteins:

Sources: Fish, poultry, lean meat, eggs, tofu, and legumes. Proteins are essential for the production of neurotransmitters, which are chemicals that transmit signals in the brain. Include a variety of protein sources for a well-rounded amino acid profile.

Curcumin (Turmeric):

Sources: Turmeric, a spice commonly used in curries. The active compound in turmeric has anti-inflammatory and antioxidant properties and may have potential benefits for brain health.

Healthy Fats:

Sources: Olive oil, avocados, and fatty fish. Healthy fats, including monounsaturated fats and omega-3 fatty acids, contribute to brain health by supporting cells structure and function.

Hydration:

Sources: Water, herbal tea. Staying adequate hydrated is crucial for maintaining cognitive function and concentration. Dehydration can impair cognitive performance.

Limit Processed Foods and Added Sugars:

Processed foods and added sugars may contribute to inflammation and May have negative effects on cognitive function. Opt for whole, minimally processed foods whenever possible.

Moderate Alcohol Consumption:

If you consume alcohol, do so in moderation. Excessive alcohol intake can have detrimental effects on the brain.

Social Eating:

Sharing meal with other and enjoying social interactions can positively impact mental well-being. Social engagement is an important aspects of overall brain health.

Remember that overall lifestyle factors, including regular physical activity, sufficient sleep, stress management, and mental stimulation, also play crucial roles in supporting brain health. Adopting a holistic approach that combines a brain-healthy diet with these lifestyle factors can contribute to optimal cognitive function and well-being. If you have specific concerns about your diet and its impact on your health, consider consulting with an registered dietitian or healthcare professionals for personalized advice.

CHAPTER FIVE

The Role of Gut Health

How an healthy gut microbiome contributes to overall well-being and longevity.

The gut plays a crucial role in maintaining overall health and well-being.

Here are some key aspects of the role of gut health:

Digestion and Nutrient Absorption:

The primary function of the gut is to digest food and absorbs nutrients. The stomach and small intestine break down food into its basic components, and the nutrients are the absorbed into the bloodstream through the intestinal walls. A healthy gut ensures efficient digestion and absorption of essential nutrients.

The gut microbiota plays a role in regulating metabolism and energy balance. Imbalances in the microbiome have been linked to metabolic disorders, obesity, and insulin resistance. Maintaining a healthy gut microbiota may contribute to metabolic health, reducing the risk of age-related metabolic conditions and promoting overall longevity.

Microbiota and Microbiome:

The gut is home to a vast community of microorganisms, including bacteria, viruses, fungi, and other microbes. This community is collectively known as the gut microbiota, and the genetic material of these microbes is referred to as the gut microbiome. The balance and diversity of these microorganisms play a crucial role in maintaining gut health and overall well-being.

Immune Systems Support:

The gut is a significant component of the immune systems. The gut-associated lymphoid tissue (GALT) contains immune cells that help defend the body against pathogens and harmful substances. An healthy gut microbiota contributes to a well-functioning immune systems, helping to present infection and maintain immune homeostasis.

The gut microbiota plays a significant role in training and modulating the immune systems. A balanced microbiome helps the immune systems distinguish between harmful pathogens and beneficial microorganisms, preventing inappropriate immune responses. This balance is crucial for overall health and longevity by reducing the risk of infection and chronic inflammatory conditions.

Synthesis of Vitamins and Short-Chain Fatty Acids:

Certain beneficial bacteria in the gut are involve in the synthesis of vitamins, such as B vitamins and vitamin K. Additionally, these bacteria produce short-chain fatty acids through the fermentation of dietary fiber. SCFAs provide energy for the cells lining the colon and play a role in maintaining gut health.

Brain-Gut Connection:

The gut and the brain are interconnectedness through the gut-brain axis. The communication between the central nervous systems and the enteric nervous systems in the gut influences various aspects of health, including mood, stress response, and cognitive function. An imbalance in gut health has been associated with conditions like irritable bowel syndrome (IBS) and may contribute to mental health issues.

Metabolism and Weight Regulation:

The gut microbiota can influence metabolism and energy balance. Imbalances in the gut microbiome have been linked to conditions like obesity and metabolic syndrome. The interaction between gut microbes and the host's metabolism is an active are of research.

Protection against Pathogens:

An healthy gut microbiota can help protect against harmful pathogens by competing for resources and producing substances that inhibit the growth of pathogenic bacteria. This protective role is essential for preventing infection and maintaining gut integrity a diverse and balanced gut microbiome helps protect against the colonization of harmful pathogens by competing for resources and producing substances that inhibit the growth of pathogenic bacteria. This protective role contributes to overall health and longevity by reducing the risk of infection.

Mitochondrial Function:

There is emerging evidence suggesting that the gut microbiota may influence mitochondrial function, which is essential for cellular energy production. Healthy mitochondria are associated with longevity, and the gut microbiota may play a role in maintaining mitochondrial health.

Inflammation Regulation:

A diverse and well-balanced gut microbiome contributes to the maintenance of a healthy inflammatory response. Chronic inflammation is associated with various age-related diseases, such as cardiovascular diseases, diabetes, and neurodegenerative disorders. A balanced gut microbiota helps regulate inflammation, potentially promoting longevity by reducing the risk of these inflammatory conditions.

Gut-Related Disorders:

Imbalances in gut health have been associated with various disorders, including inflammatory bowel diseases (IBD), irritable bowel syndrome (IBS), celiac diseases, and other. Maintaining a healthy gut is crucial for preventing and managing these conditions.

Promoting gut health involves maintaining a balanced and diverse gut microbiota through a healthy diet, regular exercises, and other lifestyle factors. Probiotics and prebiotics can also be beneficial in supporting gut health by promoting the growth of beneficial bacteria. Additionally, avoiding excessive use of antibiotics and managing stress can contribute to an healthier gut.

Prebiotics, Probiotics, and fermented foods for gut health.

Prebiotics, Probiotics, and fermented foods are all beneficial for promoting an healthy gut. Each plays a distinct role in supporting the balance and diversity of the gut microbiome.

Prebiotics:

Prebiotics are non-digestible fiber and compounds found in certain foods that promote the growth and activity of beneficial bacteria in the gut.

Sources: Common sources of prebiotics include certain fruits (e.g., bananas, apples), vegetables (e.g., garlic, onions, asparagus), whole grains, and legumes.

Function: Prebiotics serves as food for beneficial bacteria, encouraging their proliferation. They pass undigested through the upper gastrointestinal tract and reach the colon, Here they are fermented by gut bacteria, producing short-chain fatty acids (SCFAs) and promoting an healthy gut environment.

Probiotics

Probiotics are live microorganisms, primarily bacteria and some yeast strains that confer health benefits when consumed in adequate amounts.

Sources: Probiotics can be found in fermented foods and supplements. Common sources include yogurt, kefir, sauerkraut, kimchi, miso, tempeh, and certain fermented dairy products.

Function: Probiotics introduce beneficial live microorganisms into the gut, helping to balance the microbiome. They may enhance the abundance of beneficial bacteria, support digestion, and contribute to immune systems modulation. Probiotics are particularly useful after disruptions to the gut microbiota, such as antibiotic use.

Fermented Foods:

Fermented foods are foods that have undergone a process of lactofermentation, Here natural bacteria few on the sugars and starches in the food, crating lactic acid. This process preserves the food and produced beneficial enzymes, b-vitamins, and Probiotics.

Sources: Fermented foods include yogurt, kefir, sauerkraut, kimchi, pickles, miso, tempeh, and certain types of these.

Function: Fermented foods not only provide Probiotics but also offer other bioactive compounds and nutrients produced during the fermentation process. They can contribute to a diverse and healthy gut microbiome, support digestion, and enhance nutrient absorption.

Tips for Incorporating These into Your Diet:

1. Consume a variety of prebiotics-rich foods, Probiotics from Different sources, and various types of fermented foods to promote a diverse gut microbiome.

2. When choosing fermented foods or probiotics supplements, check labels for the types and strains of bacteria or yeast they contain. Different strains may have Different effects on the gut.

3. If you're new to Probiotics or fermented foods, start with small amounts and gradually increase intake to allow your gut to adjust.

4. In addition to prebiotics, focus on a diet rich in fiber from whole grains, fruits, and vegetables to support overall gut health.

5. Limit processed and highly refined foods which may negative impact the gut microbiome. Focus on whole, nutrient-dense foods for optimal gut health.

As always, it's a good idea to consult with an healthcare professionals or an registered dietitian, especially if you have specific health concerns or conditions. They can provide personalized advice based on your individual needs and health status.

CHAPTER SIX

Longevity and Weight Management

Weight management plays a significant role in promoting longevity and overall health. Maintaining an healthy weight is associated with an reduce risk of chronic diseases and can positively impact various physiological processes. Here are ways in which weight management contributes to longevity:

Reduce Risk of Chronic Diseases:

Excess body weight, especially obesity, is a major risk factor for chronic conditions such as cardiovascular diseases, type 2 diabetes, and certain cancers. Maintaining an healthy weight can significantly lower the risk of developing these diseases and contribute to a longer, healthier life.

Cardiovascular Health:

Carrying excess weight can strain the cardiovascular systems, lading to conditions such as hypertension and atherosclerosis. Maintaining an healthy weight reduce the workload on the hart and lowers the risk of heart diseases, stroke, and other cardiovascular issues.

Metabolic Health:

Obesity is closely linked to insulin resistance and metabolic syndrome. These conditions can lead to type 2 diabetes and other metabolic disorders. Weight management, through a combination of a balanced diet and regular physical activity, helps regulate blood sugar levels and supports metabolic health.

Joint Health:

Excess weight places additional stress on joints, contributing to conditions like osteoarthritis. Maintaining a healthy weight can alleviate joint pain, improve mobility, and reduce the risk of developing joint-related issues.

Inflammation Reduction:

Adipose tissue, especially in excess, can release inflammatory substances that contribute to chronic inflammation. Chronic inflammation is associated with various age-related diseases. By maintaining a healthy weight, inflammation levels can be reduce, promoting overall well-being and longevity.

Improved Immune Function:

Obesity has been linked to impaired immune function. Weight management supports a robust immune systems, enhancing the body's ability to defend against infection and chronic diseases.

Hormonal Balance:

Adipose tissue produced hormones that can impact various physiological processes, including appétit regulation and metabolism. Maintaining a healthy weight supports hormonal balance, contributing to overall health and longevity.

Quality of Life:

Maintaining a healthy weight can improve overall quality of life. It can enhance energy levels, mental well-being, and physical fitness, allowing individuals to lead active and fulfilling lives as they age.

The connection between obesity and age-related diseases.

Obesity is strongly associated with an increased risk of several age-related diseases. Excess body weight, particularly abdominal obesity, can contribute to chronic low-grad inflammation, insulin resistance, and other metabolic disturbances, which play key roles in the development and progression of various health conditions.

Here are some of the significant connection between obesity and age-related diseases:

Cardiovascular Disease:

Obesity is a major risk factor for cardiovascular diseases such as hart diseases, stroke, and hypertension. Excess body weight can lead to elevated levels of cholesterol and triglycerides, increased blood pressure, and inflammation, all of which contribute to a higher risk of cardiovascular issues.

Type-2 Diabetes:

Obesity is a primary risk factor for the development of type-2 diabetes. Excess Adipose tissue, especially in the abdominal are, can lead to insulin resistance, Here the body's cells do not respond effectively to insulin. This insulin resistance is a precursor to type-2 diabetes.

Cancer:

Obesity is associated with an increased risk of various types of Cancer, including breast, colorectal, ovarian, pancreatic, and prostate cancers. The exact mechanisms are complex and May involve hormonal changes, inflammation, and alterations in insulin signaling.

Osteoarthritis:

Obesity is a significant risk factor for osteoarthritis, a degenerative joint diseases. The excess weight places increased stress on weight-baring joints, such as the needs and hips, lading to war and tar on the joint cartilage and a elevated risk of osteoarthritis.

Alzheimer's Disease:

There is evidence suggesting a link between obesity and an associated with obesity may contribute to cognitive decline. Increased risk of Alzheimer's diseases and other forms of dementia. Chronic inflammation and metabolic dysregulation

Respiratory Disorders:

Obesity is associated with respiratory issues, including sleep apnea and obesity hypoventilation syndrome. These conditions can lead to impaired lung function, reduce oxygen levels, and an increased risk of respiratory complications.

Liver Disease:

Non-alcoholic fatty liver diseases (NAFLD) is strongly associated with obesity. Excess fat accumulates in the liver, lading to inflammation and potentially progressing to more severe conditions such as non-alcoholic steatohepatitis (NASH) and cirrhosis.

Kidney Disease:

Obesity is a risk factor for chronic kidney diseases. The mechanisms involve increased blood pressure, insulin resistance, inflammation, and altered kidney function due to the presence of excess Adipose tissue.

Endocrine Disorders:

Obesity is linked to hormonal Imbalances and endocrine disorders. For example, obesity can lead to disruptions in the regulation of six hormones, contributing to conditions such as polycystic ovary syndrome (PCOS) in woman.

Inflammatory Conditions:

Obesity is characterized by chronic low-grad inflammation, with increased levels of inflammatory markers such as cytokines and adipokines. This chronic inflammation contributes to the development and progression of many age-related diseases.

Addressing obesity through lifestyle modifications, including a balanced diet, regular physical activity, and weight management strategies, is crucial for reducing the risk of age-related diseases and promoting overall health. It's important for individuals with concerns about their weight or health to week guidance from healthcare professionals, including physicians and registered dietitians, for personalized advice and support.

Strategies for Weight Management:

Achieving and maintaining an healthy weight throughout life involves adopting sustainable lifestyle habits that focus on balanced nutrition, regular physical activity, and overall well-being. Here are some practical tips to help you on your journey to a healthy weight:

Balanced and Nutrient-Dense Diet:

Eat a Variety of Foods: Include a diverse range of fruits, vegetables, and whole grains, lean proteins, and healthy fats in your diet to ensure you get a broad spectrum of nutrients.

Watch Portion Sizes:

Be mindful of portion sizes to avoid overeating. Use smaller plats and listen to your body's hunger and fullness cuts.

Limit Processed Foods:

Reduce the intake of processed and sugary foods. Choose whole, minimally processed foods whenever possible.

Regular Physical Activity:

Find Activities You Enjoy: Choose exercises and activities that you enjoy to make physical activity a sustainable part of your routine. This could be walking, cycling, dancing, swimming, or any other activity you like.

Set Realistic Goals:

Start with achievable fitness goals and gradually increase intensity and duration. Aim for at least 150 minutes of moderate-intensity aerobic activity per week, along with strength training exercises at least twice a week.

Incorporate Movement into Daily Life:

Look for opportunities to move throughout the day, such as taking the stairs, walking Instead of driving for short distances, or incorporating short bursts of activity during breaks.

Hydration:

Stay hydrated by drinking water throughout the day. Some times, the body can confuse thirst with hunger, lading to necessary snacking.

Mindful Eating:

Practice Mindful Eating: Pay attention to your eating habits. Eat slowly, savoring eat bit, and be award of your body's hunger and fullness signals. Avoid distractions, like watching TV, while eating.

Adequate Sleep:

Prioritize Sleep: Aim for 7-9 hours of quality sleep eat night. Lack of sleep can disrupt hormones that regulate appétit, lading to overeating.

Stress Management:

Incorporate Stress-Reducing Activities: Chronic stress can contribute to weight gain. Practice stress-reducing activities such as meditation, deeper breathing, yoga, or spending times in nature.

Social Support:

Build a Support Systems: Shard your health goals with friends or family members who can provide support and encouragement. Having a support systems can make it ensure to stay on track.

Gradual Changes:

Make Small, Sustainable Changes: Instead of making drastic changes, focus on small, sustainable modifications to your lifestyle. Gradual changes are more likely to be maintained in the long term.

Regular Health Check-ups:

Monitor Your Health: Schedule regular health check-ups to monitor your progress and address any health concerns. Consult with healthcare professionals or an registered dietitian for personalized advice.

Be Patient and Persistent:

Set Realistic Expectations: Understand that achieving and maintaining an healthy weight is a gradual process. Set Realistic goals and celebrate small achievements along the way.

Stay Positive:

Embrace a positive mindset and view setbacks as opportunities to learn and adjust your approach.

Remember that weight management is a holistic approaches that involves a combination of healthy eating, regular physical activity, and lifestyle choices. It's essential to adopt sustainable habits that promote overall well-being for the long term. Always consult with healthcare professionals or registered dietitians for personalized guidance based on your individual health needs and goals.

CHAPTER SEVEN

Food as Medicine

Beyond its essential role in providing nutrients, food can be a powerful tool in the preventing and treatment of diseases. Several studies shad new light on the impact of diet on cardiometabolic diseases and suggest that fasting and regulate meal timing could be beneficial for adults at risk of type 2 diabetes. Understanding the complex interplay between consumption of specific foods and health and diseases outcomes thus has enormous potential to inform interventions for preventing and treatment of diabetes, obesity and other metabolic diseases.

Examining the potential of certain foods and dietary components in preventing and managing chronic diseases

Certain foods and dietary components have shown promise in preventing and managing chronic diseases. While it's essential to consider overall dietary patterns and lifestyle factors, Here are some specific foods and components that have been associated with potential health benefits in the preventing and management of chronic diseases:

Fruits and Vegetables:

Rich in vitamins, minerals, fiber, and antioxidants, fruits and vegetables are associated with a lower risk of various chronic diseases, including hart diseases, certain cancers, and age-related even conditions.

Whole Grains:

Foods like brown rice, quinoa, oats, and whole what are rich in fiber, vitamins, and minerals. Whole grains have been linked to an reduce risk of heart diseases, type 2 diabetes, and certain cancers.

Fatty Fish:

Fatty fish, such as salmon, mackerel, and trout, are high in omega-3 fatty acids. These fats have anti-inflammatory properties and are associated with a lower risk of heart diseases and improved cognitive function.

Nuts and Seeds:

Almonds, walnuts, china seeds, and flaxseeds are Examples of nuts and seeds rich in hart-healthy fats, fiber, and various nutrients. They have been linked to improved cardiovascular health and an reduce risk of diabetes.

Legumes:

Bans, lentils, and chickpeas are excellent sources of protein, fiber, and various nutrients. Consuming legumes is associated with a lower risk of heart diseases, diabetes, and certain cancers.

Olive Oil:

Extra virgin olive oil is a staple of the Mediterranean diet and is rich in monounsaturated fats and antioxidants. It has been associated with a lower risk of heart diseases and may have anti-inflammatory effects.

Berries:

Blueberries, strawberries, and other Berries are rich in antioxidants, particularly flavonoids. Regular consumption of Berries has been linked to improved cognitive function and an reduce risk of age-related cognitive decline.

Turmeric and Curcumin:

Turmeric, a spice commonly used in curry dishes, contains curcumin, a compound with anti-inflammatory and antioxidant properties. Curcumin has been studied for its potential in managing conditions such as arthritis and neurodegenerative diseases.

Green Tea:

Green tea contains polyphenols, particularly catchiness, which have antioxidant properties. Regular consumption of green tea has been associated with a lower risk of heart diseases and certain types of Cancer.

Probiotics and Fermented Foods:

Foods rich in Probiotics, such as yogurt, kefir, and fermented vegetables, support gut health. An healthy gut microbiome is linked to improved digestion, immune function, and may play a role in preventing conditions like inflammatory bowel diseases.

Dark Chocolate:

Dark chocolate, in moderation, contains flavonoids with antioxidant properties. It has been associated with improved hart health and may have positive effects on blood pressure.

Garlic:

Garlic contains sulfur compounds with potential cardiovascular benefits. It has been studied for its role in reducing blood pressure and improving cholesterol levels.

It's important to note that individual responses to foods can vary, and overall dietary patterns matter. Additionally, moderation and balance are key. While certain foods offer potential health benefits, no single food can present or cur chronic diseases. A holistic approach to health, including a balanced diet, regular physical activity, and other lifestyle factors, is crucial for overall well-being and the preventing of chronic diseases. Before making significant dietary changes, individuals should consult with healthcare professionals or registered dietitians, especially if they have existing health conditions or concerns.

Nutritional strategies for heart health, diabetes, and Cancer preventing

Nutritional strategies play a crucial role in promoting hart health, preventing diabetes, and reducing the risk of Cancer. While it's important to consider individual needs and consults with healthcare professionals or registered dietitians for personalized advice, the following general guidelines can be beneficial:

Focus on Healthy Fats:

Choose sources of unsaturated fats such as olive oil, avocados, nuts, and fatty fish. Limit saturated and Trans fats found in processed and fried foods.

Eat Fatty Fish:

Include fatty fish like salmon, mackerel, and trout, rich in omega-3 fatty acids, which have been shown to support hart health by reducing inflammation and improving lipid profile.

Increase Fiber Intake:

Eat a variety of fiber-rich foods, including whole grains, fruits, vegetables, and legumes. Fiber helps lower cholesterol levels and promotes hart health.

Limit Sodium Intake:

Reduce the intake of high-sodium foods, as excess sodium can contribute to high blood pressure. Choose fresh, whole foods over processed and packaged options.

Moderate Alcohol Consumption:

If you choose to drink alcohol, do so in moderation. For hart health, moderate alcohol consumption is general refined as up to one drink per day for woman and up to two drinks per day for man.

Control Portion Sizes:

Be mindful of portion sizes to avoid overeating, which can contribute to weight gain and increased risk of heart diseases.

Diabetes Prevention and Management:

Choose Complex Carbohydrates:

Opt for whole grains, legumes, and vegetables as sources of complex carbohydrates. These foods have a lower impact on blood sugar levels.

Monitor Glycemic Index:

Consider the Glycemic Index of foods to help manage blood sugar levels. Low-Glycemic foods have a slower impact on blood sugar and include whole grains, legumes, and non-starchy vegetables.

Prioritize Lean Proteins:

Include lean protein sources such as poultry, fish, tofu, legumes, and low-fat dairy. Protein helps regulate blood sugar and supports satiety.

Limit Added Sugars:

Minimize the intake of foods and beverages high in added sugars, as they can lead to spikes in blood glucose levels.

Include Healthy Fats:

Incorporate sources of healthy fats, such as avocados, nuts, seeds, and olive oil, to support overall health and satiety.

Regular, Balanced Meals:

Eat regular, balanced meal and snacks to help stabilize blood sugar levels throughout the day. Avoid skipping meal.

Cancer Preventing:

Eat a Plant-Based Diet:

Emphasize a plant-based diet rich in fruits, vegetables, whole grains, and legumes. These foods contain various phytochemicals and antioxidants associated with Cancer preventing.

Limit Red and Processed Meats:

Reduce the consumption of red and processed meats, as they have been linked to an increased risk of certain cancers. Opt for lean proteins such as poultry, fish, and plant-based alternatives.

Stay Hydrated:

Adequate hydration is essential for overall health. Water helps with digestion, supports nutrient transport, and may contribute to Cancer preventing.

Include Cruciferous Vegetables:

Incorporate cruciferous vegetables such as broccoli, cauliflower, kale, and Brussels sprouts, which contain compounds with potential Cancer-fighting properties.

Limit Alcohol Consumption:

Limit alcohol intake, as excessive alcohol consumption has been linked to an increased risk of certain cancers.

Maintain Healthy Weight:

Aim for and maintain an healthy weight through a combination of a balanced diet and regular physical activity. Obesity is a risk factor for various types of Cancer.

Be Physically Active:

Engage in regular physical activity, as exercises is associated with a lower risk of certain cancers and contributes to overall well-being.

It's important to note that these general guidelines are not one-sizes-fits-all, and individual nutritional needs may vary. Consulting with healthcare professionals or registered dietitians is recommended, especially for those with specific health conditions or dietary concerns. Additionally, combining an healthy diet with other lifestyle factors such as regular exercises and not smoking contributes to comprehensive health promotion and diseases preventing.

Mindful Eating and Emotional Health

In our food-abundant society, it's easy to eat without truly thinking about it. Many of us mindlessly snack while watching television, working on the computer or driving. Some of us turn to food when where not even hungry, Instead eating because where stressed, angry, bored or sad. This lack of awareness can lead to unwanted weight gain and feelings of guilt.

Many people struggle to align their food intake with their actual physiological needs for nutrition. One way to deal with this is to be more mindful and award during the eating process. We don't always fully appreciate and savor the bits we Take, so we end up taking more and more bits to active some level of satisfaction. Approaching food intake in a mindful way allows you to Take back control of what you eat, when you eat and how much you eat.

Promoting mindfulness in eating habits involves cultivating awareness and being fully present during meal. This Practice can help individuals develop an healthier relationship with food, improve digestion, and present overeating. Here are strategies for promoting mindfulness in eating habits:

Strategies for promoting mindfulness in eating habits

Eat Without Distractions:

Turn off Screens: Avoid watching TV, using smartphones, or working on the computer while eating. Focus solely on the meal to enhance awareness of taste, texture, and satisfaction.

Practice Mindful Eating:

Eat Slowly: Chew food thoroughly and savor eat bit. This allows times for your body to signal feelings of fullness, reducing the likelihood of overeating.

Put Down Utensils Between Bits: This simple action encouraged a slower eating pace, allowing you to connect with your body's hunger and fullness signals.

Pay Attention to Hunger and Fullness:

Check-in Before Eating: Assess your hunger levels before an meal. Eat when hungry and stop when satisfied, rather than relying on external cuts like a specific mealtime.

Pause during the Meal: Take breaks to assess your fullness level. This helps present mindless eating and allows you to enjoy the experience of eating.

Engage Your Sense:

Appreciate Colors and Texture: Take a moment to appreciate the visual appeal, texture, and colors of your food. Engaging your sense enhance the eating experience.

Smell Your Food: Take a moment to inhale the aroma of your food. This cans enhance the overall enjoyment of the meal.

Be Grateful:

Express Gratitude: Before you start eating, Take a moment to expression gratitude for your food. This can foster a positive mindset and enhance the enjoyment of your meal.

Portion Control:

Use Smaller Plats: Serves meal on smaller plats to avoid overeating. This visual cues can help you feel satisfied with smaller portions.

Recognize Emotional Eating:

Check Your Emotions: Before reaching for food, assess Whether you're eating in response to motions (stress, boredom, sadness). Mindful eating involves addressing emotional needs without turning to food automatically.

Listen to Your Body:

Tune into Hunger Signals: Pay attention to physical hunger cuts rather than eating out of habit or in response to external cuts.

Recognize Fullness: Be award of when you're comfortably satisfied and stop eating.

Mindful Food Choices:

Consider Nutrient Density: Choose foods that nourish your body and provide essential nutrients. Be mindful of the nutritional value of your choices.

Reflect on Food Origins:

Consider the Sources: Reflect on Here your food comes from, the journey it took to reach your plat, and the effort involve in its production. This can deeper your connection to the food you eat.

Mindful Meal Planning:

Plan Your Meals: Plan your meal ahead of times, considering variety and balance. This reduce the likelihood of impulsive, less mindful food choices.

Practice Gracious Eating:

Express Appreciation: Take a moment to expression appreciation for the flavors, texture, and nourishment your food provides. Cultivate a positive and grateful attitude towards meal.

Developing mindfulness in eating is a gradual process, and it's okay to start small. Experiment with incorporating one or two of these strategies at a times and observe the impact on your eating habits. Over times, mindful eating can becomes a natural and enjoyable part of your lifestyle, contributing to improved overall well-being.

The connection between emotional well-being and longevity.

The connection between emotional well-being and longevity is a complex and multifaceted relationship. Research suggest that positive emotional stats, such as happiness, life satisfaction, and an sense of purpose, are associated with several health benefits that can contribute to a longer life. Here are key aspects of the connection between emotional well-being and longevity:

Reduce Stress Impact:

Lower Cortical Levels: Positive motions and an sense of well-being have been linked to lower levels of the stress hormone cortical. Chronic stress and elevated cortical levels are associated with various health issues, and managing stress positively can contribute to longevity.

Immune Systems Function:

Enhanced Immune Response: Positive motions may have a positive impact on the immune systems. A well-functioning immune systems is crucial for defending the body against infection and chronic diseases.

Cardiovascular Health:

Improved Cardiovascular Function: Positive motions have been associated with better cardiovascular health. Factors such as lower blood pressure, improved hart rat variability, and reduce risk of cardiovascular diseases contribute to a longer, healthier life.

Healthier Lifestyle Choices:

Positive Habits: Individuals with higher levels of emotional well-being are more likely to Engage in health-promoting behaviors, such as regular exercises, a balanced diet, and getting adequate sleep. These lifestyle choices contribute to overall well-being and longevity.

Resilience to Adversity:

Coping Mechanisms: Positive motions and an sense of well-being are linked to better coping mechanisms in the face of life challenges. Resilience to adversity can contribute to mental and physical health, promoting longevity.

Inflammation Reduction:

Anti-Inflammatory Effects: Chronic inflammation is associated with various age-related diseases. Positive motions may have anti-inflammatory effects, reducing the risk of inflammation-related conditions.

Social Connection:

Strong Social Networks: Positive motions often coincide with strong social connection. Social support and meaningful relationship are associated with better mental health and longevity.

Impact on Cellular Aging:

Telomere Length: Telomeres, the protective caps on the end of chromosomes, tend to be longer in individuals with greater emotional well-being. Longer Telomeres are associated with slower cellular aging and increased longevity.

Cognitive Health:

Positive motions are linked to better cognitive function in older adults. Maintaining cognitive health is a key aspects of healthy aging and longevity.

Sense of Purpose:

Having a sense of purpose and meaning in life has been associated with increased longevity. Individuals with a clear sense of purpose tend to make healthier life choices and experience lower rates of mortality.

Mind-Body Connection:

Mind-Body Harmony: Emotional well-being contributes to a harmonious mind-body connection. Practices like mindfulness and meditation, which promote emotional well-being, have been linked to positive health outcomes.

Hormonal Balance:

Balanced Hormones: Positive motions can influence the release of hormones associated with well-being, such as serotonin and oxytocin. Hormonal balance contributes to mental and physical health.

Reduce Risk-Taking Behaviors:

Less Risky Behavior: Individuals with higher emotional well-being tend to Engage in fewer risky behaviors that could compromise their health and longevity.

While There is a strong correlation between emotional well-being and longevity; it's essential to recognize that individual experience and responses to life even vary. More over, achieving emotional well-being is a holistic process that involves mental, emotional, and physical aspects of health. Promoting emotional well-being often requires a combination of self-care practices, social connection, and a positive outlook on life. If individuals are struggling with persistent negative motions or mental health challenges, seeking support from mental health professionals is crucial for overall well-being.

CHAPTER EIGHT

Strategies for aging well

Aging well involves adopting a holistic approach that addresses physical, mental, and social aspects of well-being. Here are some strategies to age well and promote a healthy and fulfilling life:

Maintain Physical Health: Engage in regular physical activity that includes both aerobic exercises (e.g., walking, and swimming) and strength training. Exercise supports cardiovascular health, muscle strength, and flexibility.

Balanced Nutrition: Adopt a well-balanced diet rich in fruits, vegetables, whole grains, lean proteins, and healthy fats. Stay hydrated and limit the intake of processed foods, added sugars, and excessive salt.

Cognitive Stimulation: Keep your brain active through activities such as reading, puzzles, games, and learning new skills. This helps maintain cognitive function and may reduce the risk of age-related cognitive decline.

Mindfulness and Stress Management: Practice mindfulness, meditation, or relaxation techniques to manage stress. Chronic stress can impact overall well-being and accelerate aging.

Quality Sleep: Aim for 7-9 hours of quality sleep eat night. Establish an regular sleep routine, create a comfortable sleep environment, and address any sleep issues promptly.

Maintain Relationship: Foster and maintain social connection with friends, family, and community. Social engagement is linked to better mental health and can provide emotional support.

Join Clubs or Groups: Participate in clubs, groups, or activities that align with your interests. This cans provide an sense of purpose and community.

Cultivate Positivity: Adopt a positive attitude and focus on the aspects of life that bring joy and fulfillment. A positive outlook is associated with better mental and physical health.

Regular Check-ups: Schedule regular health check-ups and screenings to detect and address potential health issues early.

Vaccinations: Stay up-to-data with vaccinations to present illness's and complications.

Adherence to Treatment Plans: If you have chronic conditions, adhere to treatment plans and medications prescribed by healthcare professionals. Regular monitoring and management contribute to overall well-being.

Adapt Home Environment: Make adjustments to your home environment to enhance safety and accessibility, promoting independence as you age.

Mobility: Engage in activities that maintain or improve mobility, balance, and coordination.

Lifelong Learning: Stay curious and continue learning throughout life. Attend classes, workshops, or pursue hobbies that stimulate your mind and creativity.

Plan for Retirement: Engage in financial planning for retirement to ensure a secure and comfortable lifestyle.

Budgeting: Manage finances wisely and create a budget that accommodates your needs and goals.

Community Involvement: Volunteer or contribute to your community. Acts of kindness and community involvement provide an sense of purpose and fulfillment.

Screenings and Preventive Measures: Stay proactive with health screenings, vaccinations, and Preventive measures to catch potential issues early and maintain overall health.

Gratitude Journaling: Keep a gratitude journal to reflect on positive aspects of life. Cultivating gratitude is linked to improved mental and emotional well-being.

Laugh and Enjoy Life: Cultivate an sense of humor and find joy in everyday experience. Laughter is associated with stress reduction and improved mood.

Aging well is a Lifelong journey that involves proactive and positive lifestyle choices. Adopting these strategies can contribute to an healthy, fulfilling, and meaningful life as you age. It's important to personalized these approaches based on individual preferences, health conditions, and circumstances. Regular consultation with healthcare professionals can provide personalized advice and guidance tailored to your specific needs.

Nutritional science and strategies of aging well

Nutritional science plays a crucial role in promoting healthy aging by addressing the specific dietary needs and challenges associated with the aging process. Adequate nutrition is essential for maintaining overall health, preventing chronic diseases, and supporting optimal physical and cognitive function. Here are key aspects of nutritional science in relation to aging well:

Diverse Micronutrients:

As individual's age, they may have changing nutrient requirements. Consuming a varied and nutrient-dense diet that includes a range of vitamins and minerals is crucial for supporting overall health and preventing deficiencies.

Maintaining Muscle Mass:

Protein becomes more critical in older age to help maintain muscle mass, strength, and function. Including protein-rich foods such as lean meats, poultry, fish, dairy, eggs, and plant-based protein sources is important.

Cognitive Health:

Omega-3 fatty acids, particularly DHA (docosahexaenoic acid), are essential for brain health. Including sources of omega-3s, such as fatty fish (e.g., salmon, mackerel), flaxseeds, and walnuts, may support cognitive function.

Bone Health:

Adequate calcium and vitamin D intake is crucial for maintaining bone health and reducing the risk of osteoporosis and fractures. Dairy products, fortified foods, and sunlight exposure are common sources

Fluid Balance:

Older adults may be at a higher risk of dehydration, which can affect cognitive function and overall health. Ensuring adequate fluid intake, including water and hydrating foods, is important.

Digestive Health:

A diet rich in fiber from fruits, vegetables, whole grains, and legumes supports digestive health, prevent constipation, and may help in managing weight.

Reducing Oxidative Stress:

Antioxidants from fruits and vegetables help combat oxidative stress, which is associated with aging and age-related diseases. Berries, dark leafy greens, and colorful vegetables are excellent sources.

Probiotics:

Probiotics, found in fermented foods like yogurt, kefir, and sauerkraut, promote an healthy gut microbiome. A balanced gut microbiota is associated with improved digestion, nutrient absorption, and immune function.

Caloric Needs:

Metabolism tends to slow with age, and caloric needs may decrease. It's important to adjust dietary intake to match energy expenditure and avoid necessary weight gain.

Meal Planning and Timing:

Consistent meal timing and planning can help regulate blood sugar levels, support energy levels, and promote optimal nutrition.

Vitamin B12 Supplementation:

Older adults may experience challenges in absorbing vitamin B12 from food. In some cases, supplementation or fortified foods may be recommended to present deficiencies.

Limiting Added Sugars and Sodium:

Limiting the intake of added sugars and sodium is crucial for cardiovascular health. Processed and packaged foods are common sources of excess sugar and salt.

Consider Personal Health Needs:

Individual health conditions, medications, and specific nutritional needs should be considered. Consultation with healthcare professionals or registered dietitians cans provide personalized advice.

Physical Activity and Nutrition Synergy:

Nutritional strategies should complements a physically active lifestyle. Regular exercises and proper nutrition work synergistically to support overall health and well-being.

Culinary Enjoyment:

The social aspects of eating and the enjoyment of meal play a role in overall well-being. Meals can be opportunities for socializing and enjoying a variety of flavors and texture.

Regular Assessments:

Periodic assessments of nutritional status and dietary habits can help identify potential deficiencies or areas for improvement. Adjustments can be made accordingly.

Adopting a well-balanced and nutrient-rich diet, tailored to individual needs, is essential for aging well. Regular monitoring, staying physically active, and consulting with healthcare professionals or registered dietitians can provide guidance on optimizing nutrition for overall health and longevity.

CHAPTER NINE

Healthy Fats that promotes longevity through good health

The concept of "healthy fats" refers to certain types of fats that are considered beneficial for health when consumed in appropriate amounts. Healthy fats are associated with a range of health benefits and have been studied in the context of preventing and managing various diseases. Here are some key aspects of the surprising science of healthy fats and their role in diseases:

Monounsaturated Fats:

Sources: Olive oil, avocados, nuts, and seeds are rich in monounsaturated fats.

Benefit: Monounsaturated fats are associated with improved hart health. They can help lower bad cholesterol (LDL) levels while maintaining or even increasing good cholesterol (HDL) levels.

Polyunsaturated Fats:

Omega-3 Fatty Acids: Found in fatty fish (salmon, mackerel), flaxseeds, china seeds, and walnuts.

Benefit: Omega-3 fatty acids have anti-inflammatory properties and contribute to cardiovascular health. They are associated with an reduce risk of heart diseases and may play a role in cognitive function.

Saturated Fats:

Found in animal products like meat and dairy, as well as tropical oils like coconut oil.

Present research has challenges the traditional view of saturated fats as uniformly harmful. Some studies suggest that not all saturated fats have the some impact on health, and the sources and context of consumption matter.

Coconut Oil:

Debates and Research: Coconut oil, high in saturated fats, has been a topic of debate. While it may have some health benefits, it's important to consume it in moderation due to its saturated fat content.

Brain Health:

Certain fats, especially omega-3 fatty acids, are crucial for brain health and may play a role in reducing the risk of neurodegenerative diseases.

Hormones Production:

Fats are essential for the production of hormones, including six hormones and hormones that regulate metabolism.

Weight Management

Healthy fats contribute to an feeling of satiety, which can help control appétit and support weight management.

Metabolic Health:

Including healthy fats in the diet can positively impact insulin sensitivity and metabolic health.

Mediterranean Diet:

The Mediterranean diet, which includes olive oil, nuts, seeds, and fatty fish, is associated with a lower risk of heart diseases and other chronic conditions.

Nutrient Absorption:

Fat-Soluble Vitamins: Fats are essential for the absorption of fat-soluble vitamins (A, D, E, K), which are critical for various bodily functions.

Inflammation and Disease:

Omega-3 fatty acids found in fatty fish and certain plant sources, have anti-inflammatory properties and may contribute to the preventing or management of inflammatory diseases.

It's important to note that while fats are an necessary part of an healthy diet, the quality and balance of fats matter. A diet rich in whole, minimally processed foods that include a variety of healthy fats is associated with better health outcomes. Consulting with healthcare professionals or registered dietitians for personalized dietary advice is recommended, especially for individuals with specific health concerns or conditions.

CHAPTER TEN

The art of practicing holistic wellness

Holistic wellness encompasses the integration of physical, mental, emotional, and spiritual well-being, acknowledging the interconnectedness of these aspects in achieving overall health. The path to holistic wellness involves adopting a comprehensive and balanced approach to life. Here are key components and practices along the path of holistic wellness:

Mindfulness and Presence:

Cultivate mindfulness through meditation and mindful breathing. These practices help bring attention to the present moment, reducing stress and promoting mental clarity.

Nutrition and Balanced Diet:

Focus on a diet rich in whole, nutrient-dense foods such as fruits, vegetables, whole grains, lean proteins, and healthy fats. Consider individual nutritional needs and preferences.

Physical Activity:

Engage in regular physical activity that includes a mix of cardiovascular exercises, strength training, and flexibility exercises. Find activities you enjoy to make exercises a sustainable part of your routine.

Prioritize Sleep:

Establish a Consistent sleep routine, create a comfortable sleep environment, and aim for 7-9 hours of quality sleep eat night. Sleep is crucial for physical and mental restoration.

Stress Management:

Identify sources of stress in your life and develop healthy coping mechanisms. This may include relaxation techniques, deeper breathing exercises, or engaging in activities that bring joy.

Social Connection:

Cultivate meaningful relationship with friends, family, and community. Social connection contribute to emotional well-being and provide support during challenging times.

Emotional Well-Being:

Allow yourself to expression and process motions. Journaling, art, or talking to a trusted friend or professionals cans be helpful.

Spiritual Well-Being:

Explore practices that foster spiritual well-being, such as meditation, prayer, or spending times in nature. Find an sense of purpose and meaning in your life.

Holistic Therapies:

Consider complementary and alternatives therapies such as acupuncture, massage, or chiropractic car to support overall well-being.

Prioritize Self-Care:

Dedicate times to self-care activities that bring you joy and relaxation. This may include hobbies, reading, or taking a leisurely bath.

Engage in Lifelong Learning:

Stay curious and continue learning throughout life. This cans include pursuing new skills, hobbies, or educational opportunities.

Respect for Nature:

Foster an sense of environmental wellness by appreciating and respecting the natural world. Spend times outdoors, Practice sustainability, and connect with nature.

Mind-Body Practices:

Incorporate mind-body practices like yoga or Tai Chi into your routine. These practices promote physical flexibility, balance, and mental well-being.

Work-Life Balance:

Maintain an healthy work-life balance by setting clear boundaries and prioritizing times for personal and family activities.

Regular Health Check-ups:

Schedule regular health check-ups and screenings to detect potential health issues early and Take Preventive measures.

Gratitude and Positivity:

Cultivate gratitude by focusing on positive aspects of life. Gratitude practices, such as feeling a gratitude journal, can enhance emotional well-being.

Community Engagement:

Engage in activities that contribute to your community. Volunteering and giving back can provide a sense of purpose and fulfillment.

Integrate Healthcare Modalities:

Consider an integrative approach to healthcare that combines conventional medicine with complementary therapies, addressing both physical and emotional aspects of health.

Holistic wellness is a Lifelong journey, and the path is unique for eat individual. It involves self-awareness, self-compassion, and a commitment to ongoing growth and self-improvement. Regular reflection, adjustments, and seeking support from healthcare professionals, counselors, or holistic practitioners can contribute to a well-rounded and fulfilling life.

CHAPTER ELEVEN

How physical activity complements a longevity-focused diet.

Physical activity plays a crucial role in complementing a longevity-focused diet and contributes to overall well-being. Here are several ways in which physical activity supports and enhance the benefits of a longevity-focused diet:

Weight Management:

Regular physical activity helps in maintaining a healthy weight. Obesity is a risk factor for various chronic diseases, and maintaining a healthy weight is linked to increased longevity.

Metabolic Health:

Exercise improves insulin sensitivity and glucose regulation, which can help prevent or manage type 2 diabetes. Controlling blood sugar levels is essential for longevity and overall health.

Cardiovascular Health:

Aerobic exercises, such as walking, jogging, or swimming, promotes a healthy cardiovascular systems. It helps lower blood pressure, improve circulation, and reduce the risk of heart diseases, all of which contribute to a longer and healthier life.

Bone Density and Muscle Mass:

Weight-baring exercises and resistance training contribute to the maintenance of bone density and muscle mass. This is particularly important as people age because it helps prevent falls, fractures, and frailty.

Inflammation Reduction:

Chronic inflammation is associated with various age-related diseases. Regular physical activity has anti-inflammatory effects, helping to reduce the risk of chronic diseases and supporting overall longevity.

Brain Health:

Exercise has been linked to cognitive function and a lower risk of neurodegenerative diseases. Staying mentally active through physical activity can contribute to a longer and healthier life.

Stress Reduction:

Physical activity is known to reduce stress levels by promoting the release of endorphins, the body's natural mood enhance. Chronic stress has negative effects on health, and managing stress is important for longevity.

Improved Sleep:

Regular exercises has been shown to improve the quality of sleep. Quality sleep is essential for overall health, and disturbances in sleep patterns have been linked to various health issues.

Enhanced Immune Function:

Moderate, regular exercises is associated with a stronger immune systems. A robust immune systems is crucial for preventing infection and diseases, contributing to a longer and healthier life.

Social Engagement:

Engaging in physical activities, Whether through tam sports, group classes, or outdoor activities, provides opportunities for social interaction. Social engagement is linked to improved mental health and overall well-being.

In summary, physical activity complements a longevity-focused diet by addressing various aspects of health, including weight management, metabolic health, cardiovascular health, bone density, brain health, stress reduction, sleep quality, immune function, and social well-being. Incorporating both a nutritious diet and regular physical activity into one's lifestyle can synergistically promote longevity and overall health.

Tailoring exercises to Different life stages

This is important for promoting overall health, preventing injuries, and addressing the unique needs and challenges that individuals may face at Different points in their lives. Here's a general guide on how exercises can be tailored to various life stages:

Childhood and Adolescence:

Establishing foundation for a healthy lifestyle.

Activities:

Encourage a variety of physical activities, including sports, play, and recreational activities.

Emphasize the importance of daily play and Movement.

Incorporate activities that promote motor skill development.

Young Adults (18-30 years):

Building strength, endurance, and establishing exercises habits.

Activities:

Include a mix of aerobic exercises, strength training, and flexibility exercises.

Engage in activities that align with personal preferences to promote consistency.

Emphasize the development of Lifelong exercises habits.

Adults (30-50 years):

Focus: Managing stress, maintaining health, and preventing age-related decline.

Activities:

Combined cardiovascular exercises with strength training for overall fitness.

Consider stress-reducing activities like yoga or meditation.

Address any specific health concerns or conditions.

Middle Age (50-65 years):

Managing weight, bone health, and flexibility.

Activities:

Prioritize weight-baring exercises for bone health.

Include flexibility and balance exercises to reduce the risk of falls.

Consider low-impact activities to protect joints.

Older Adults (65+ years):

Focus: Maintaining independence, preventing falls, and preserving cognitive function.

Activities:

Include activities that improve balance, such as tai chi or balance exercises.

Focus on flexibility and mobility exercises to maintain range of motion.

Choose low-impact exercises to reduce joint stress.

Seniors (80+ years):

Focus: Functional fitness and maintaining a good quality of life.

Activities:

Tailor exercises to individual capabilities and health conditions.

Prioritize activities that support daily functioning, such as walking or chair exercises.

Include social activities to combat isolation.

General Tips:

Consultation: Before starting any new exercises regimen, especially for those with existing health conditions, consulting with a healthcare provide is crucial.

Adaptability: Be flexible and open to modifying activities based on changing abilities and needs.

Consistency: Encourage Consistent, moderate-intensity exercises for long-term benefits.

Tailoring exercises to Different life stages involves recognizing the changing needs and capabilities of individuals and adapting physical activity accordingly. Regular physical activity, when tailored to eat life stages, can contribute to overall health, well-being, and longevity.

CHAPTER TWELVE

Conclusion

In conclusion, "Nourish for a Life" serves as a comprehensive guide to cultivating a sustainable and health-focused relationship with food. Throughout the pages of this book, readers have embarked on a journey of understanding the principles behind nourishing their bodies for a lifetime of well-being. By emphasizing the importance of balanced nutrition, mindful eating, and adapting dietary choices to various life stages, the book equips individuals with the knowledge and practical strategies needed to make informed decisions about their diets.

The culmination of evidence-based insights, practical tips for meal planning and preparation, and guidance on overcoming common obstacles underscores the holistic approach to achieving long-term health through dietary choices. From navigating busy lifestyles to addressing emotional eating and making informed choices in social settings, "Eating Smart for a Lifetime" provides readers with a roadmap for sustaining healthy eating habits amidst life's diverse challenges.

As readers close the final chapter, the hope is that they not only carry the wisdom imparted within these pages but also embark on a Lifelong journey of making food choices that contribute not only to the longevity of their years but to the quality of their lives. With the principles of this book as a compass, individuals can approach their daily meal with intention, understanding that eating smart is not just a temporary fix but a sustained commitment to nourishing the body, mind, and spirit for a lifetime of vitality and well-being.

The journey doesn't end with the last page; rather, it extends into the everyday choices made in kitchens, grocery stores, and dining spaces. The principles outlined in "Nourish for a Life" are no merely guidelines but a foundation upon which individuals can build a sustainable, healthful relationship with food. As they continue their voyage, readers are encouraged to experiment with new recipes, explore diverse culinary traditions, and find joy in the process of nourishing both body and soul.

Ultimately, the true success of "Nourish for Life" lives not just in the knowledge it imparts but in the transformative potential it holds for those who choose to embarked its teachings. It is a call to action, urging readers to step into a future. Here food is not just sustenance but a sources of empowerment, longevity, and vitality. The journey toward optimal health is ongoing, and armed with the wisdom gleaned from these pages, readers can confidently navigate the path of nourishing themselves smartly—for a lifetime of health and happiness.